# The Complete Ketogenic Diet:

## Your Complete Guide to Living the Keto Lifestyle

The Simple, Easy Way To Start The Ketogenic Diet

Linden Hale

Ketogenic Diet

# Ketogenic Diet

# The Complete Ketogenic Diet:

# Your Complete Guide to Living the Keto Lifestyle

The Simple, Easy Way To Start The Ketogenic Diet

Linden Hale

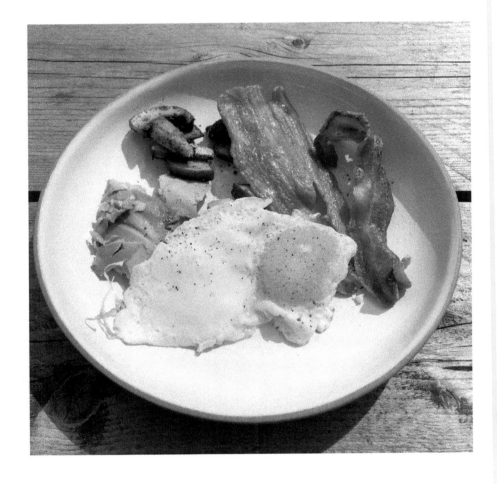

# What is the ketogenic diet?

The ketogenic diet is a nutritional strategy based on the reduction of dietary carbohydrates, which "forces" the body to produce autonomously the glucose necessary for survival and to increase the energy consumption of fats contained in adipose tissue.

Ketogenic diet means "diet that produces ketone bodies" (a metabolic residue of energy production).

Regularly produced in minimal amounts and easily disposed of by urine and pulmonary ventilation, in the ketogenic diet ketone bodies reach a level higher than the normal condition. The undesirable excess of ketone bodies, responsible for the tendency to lower blood pH, is called ketosis.

Motor activity also affects, positively or negatively (as appropriate), the condition of ketoacidosis.

The presence of ketone bodies in the blood exerts different effects on the body; some are considered useful in the slimming process, others are "collateral".

There is not only one type of ketogenic diet and all the eating styles that provide a lower quantity of calories, carbohydrates and sometimes proteins than necessary are ketogenic; low carb and potentially ketogenic are certainly the Atkins diet and the LCHF (low carb, high fat).

Some types of ketogenic diets are used in the clinical field (for example against epilepsy not responsive to drugs, severe obesity associated with certain metabolic pathologies, etc.), but these systems are mainly used in the field of fitness and aesthetic culture.

More:Low Carb Diets

Characteristics of the ketogenic diet
The ketogenic diet (in English ketogenic diet or keto diet) is a nutritional scheme:
Low in calories (low-calorie diet)
Low percentage and absolute content of carbohydrates (low carb diet)
High percentage content of proteins, even if the absolute quantity (in grams) is more often medium - remember that neoglucogenic amino acids can be used by the liver to produce glucose
High percentage content of lipids.
Protocol
What to eat in the ketogenic diet?
The most important aspect to reach the state of ketosis is to eat foods that do not contain carbohydrates, limit those that provide little of them and avoid foods that are rich in them.
Recommended foods are:
Meat, fishery products and eggs - Basic food group I
Cheeses - Fundamental food group II
Fats and oils for seasoning - Fundamental food group V
Vegetables - VI and VII fundamental food groups.
Foods not recommended instead are:

Cereals, potatoes and their derivatives - Fundamental food group III

Legumes - IV fundamental group of foods

Fruits - VI and VII fundamental group of foods

Sweet drinks, various sweets, beer etc.

In general, it is recommended to maintain a carbohydrate intake less than or equal to 50 g/day, ideally organized in 3 servings with 20 g each.

A rather strict guideline for a proper ketogenic diet involves an energy breakdown of:

10% from carbohydrates

15-25% from proteins (not forgetting that proteins, as they also contain glucogenic amino acids, are involved in sustaining blood glucose levels)

70% or more from fat.

How to understand to be in ketosis?

To identify a possible state of ketosis you can perform urine tests (with special urine strips), blood tests (blood ketone meters) or breath tests (breath ketone analyzer). However, you can also rely on certain "telltale" symptoms that don't require any testing:

Dry mouth and feeling thirsty

Increased diuresis (due to acetoacetate filtration)

Acetonic breath or sweat (due to the presence of acetone) escaping through our breath

Reduced appetite

Lassitude.

How many ketones must be present in the blood? There is no real distinction between ketosis and non-ketosis. The level of these compounds is influenced by diet and lifestyle. However, it is possible to say that there is an optimal range for the proper functioning of the ketogenic diet:

Below 0.5 mmol of ketones per liter of blood is not considered ketosis.

Between 0.5-1.5 mmol/l we talk about light ketosis

With 1.5-3 mmol/l ketosis is defined as optimal

Values of more than 3 mmol/l, besides not being more effective, compromise the state of health (especially in case of diabetes mellitus type 1)

Values over 8-10 mmol/l are difficult to achieve with the diet. They are sometimes obtained in disease or by inadequate physical activity; they correlate with even very severe symptoms.

# Ketogenic Diet

# How does the ketogenic diet work?

The working mechanism of the ketogenic diet is based on the reduction of calories and dietary carbohydrates which, in association with a proper level of proteins and a high percentage of fats, should improve lipolysis and cellular lipid oxidation, therefore the total consumption of fats optimizing weight loss. The production of ketone bodies, which must be absolutely controlled, has the function of moderating the stimulus of appetite - due to their anorectic effect.

Ketogenic Metabolism

Notes on energy production

The cellular energy production takes place thanks to the metabolization of some substrates, mainly glucose and fatty acids. Mostly, this process begins in the cytoplasm (anaerobic glycolysis - without oxygen) and ends in the mitochondria (Krebs cycle - with oxygen - and ATP recharge). Note: muscle cells are also able to oxidize good quantities of branched amino acids. However, two fundamental aspects must be stressed:

Some tissues, such as nervous tissue, function "almost" exclusively on glucose

The correct cellular utilization of fatty acids is dependent on the presence of glucose that, if lacking, is produced by the liver through neoglucogenesis (starting from substrates such as glucogenic amino acids and glycerol).

Note: alone, neoglucogenesis is not able to satisfy definitively, in the long term, the metabolic demands of the entire organism.

That's why carbohydrates, even if they can't be defined as "essential", must be considered indispensable nutrients and it's recommended a minimum intake of 180 g/day (the minimum amount to ensure the full functionality of the central nervous system).

Residual ketone bodies

Let us now explain how the liberation of ketone bodies occurs.

During energy production, fatty acids are first reduced to CoA (coenzyme A) and, soon after, made to enter the Krebs cycle. Here they bind to oxaloacetate and undergo further oxidation, ending with the release of carbon dioxide and water. When the production of acetyl CoA by lipolysis exceeds the uptake capacity of oxaloacetate, the formation of so-called ketone bodies occurs.

Note: each ketone body is formed by two molecules of acetyl CoA.

Types of ketone bodies

Ketone bodies are of three types:

Acetone

Acetoacetate

3-Hydroxybutyrate.

Disposal of ketone bodies

Ketone bodies can be further oxidized, in particular by muscle cells, by the heart and to a lesser extent by the brain (which uses them mainly in glucose deficiency), or eliminated with urine and pulmonary ventilation. Needless to say that increasing ketone bodies in the blood also increases the workload of the kidneys.

If the production of ketone bodies exceeds the body's ability to dispose of them, they accumulate in the blood, resulting in the so-called ketosis.

Ketosis, ketoacidosis and metabolic acidosis
Also called ketoacidosis, this condition lowers the blood pH defining the typical picture of metabolic acidosis (typical of untreated diabetics). In extreme cases, acidosis can lead to coma and even death.

Motor activity and ketoacidosis
The role of motor activity on ketoacidosis is, in a sense, contradictory. Starting from the assumption that recourse to the ketogenic diet is in any case a metabolic forcing - which in the long run can lead to unpleasant consequences, even in a young and well-trained organism - it is necessary to specify that:

On the one hand, intense physical exercise increases the energy demands of glucose favoring the production and accumulation of ketone bodies.

On the other hand, moderate physical exercise increases the oxidation of ketone bodies themselves, opposing their accumulation and the negative effects they can exert in the body.

For further information:Example of Ketogenic Diet for Muscle Definition in Body-Building

Neoglucogenesis
We have already said that the organism needs glucose anyway and that, if it is not taken with the diet, it must be produced through neoglucogenesis. Essential for the correct functioning of nervous tissue, glucose is also necessary for the completion of lipid oxidation.

Gluconeogenesis is a process that leads to the formation of glucose starting from the carbonaceous skeleton of some amino acids (called glucogenic, or that give rise to oxaloacetate); to a lesser extent, also from glycerol and lactic acid. This process ensures a constant supply of energy even in conditions of glucose deficiency, but forces the liver and kidneys to work harder to eliminate nitrogen.

Uses

Application of the ketogenic diet

This dietary strategy is mainly used in three contexts (very different from each other):

Weight loss (better if under medical supervision)

Dietary therapy of certain metabolic pathologies such as chronic hyperglycemia, hypertriglyceridemia (only under medical control), arterial hypertension and metabolic syndrome (never in the presence of pathologies or suffering of the liver and/or kidneys)

Reduction of symptoms associated with childhood epilepsy (only when the subject does not respond to drug therapy and only under medical supervision).

Example Daily Menu

Example of daily menu of the ketogenic diet

Some examples of daily menu of ketogenic diet are reported in the article: "Ketogenic Diet Example"

More:Ketogenic Diet Example

Weekly Menu Scheme

Weekly menu scheme of ketogenic diet

For more information about the weekly menu plan of the ketogenic diet we refer you to a dedicated article: "Example of Ketogenic Diet".

More:Sample Ketogenic Diet

Results in 21 days of ketogenic diet
As we said, there are different types of ketogenic diet and not all of them offer the same results.

More:Mayo Ketogenic Diet Example

This is because, regardless of personal aptitude, the ketogenic diet is a system that requires rather careful control and monitoring. What's more, it can't (or rather, shouldn't) be protracted for too long. About 3 weeks, or 21 days, are generally well tolerated.

For this, a book entitled "21-Day Ketogenic Diet Weight Loss Challenge: Recipes and Workouts for a Slimmer, Healthier You" was produced and published. The text contains a hundred recipes and the entire food management for the dedicated period, and various workout protocols to facilitate weight loss while maintaining as much muscle mass as possible.

Needless to dwell on the evaluation of this method; as anticipated, the ketogenic diet is a rather delicate system and not to be underestimated. It is therefore impossible to standardize this method for the entire population. Leaving the full management of the ketogenic diet to consumers is wrong, because it is easily misleading. This does not mean that it does not work, but rather that it does not represent an adequate solution.

Benefits

Advantages of the ketogenic diet

The ketogenic diet can exert advantages:

It facilitates weight loss through:

Reduction of total calories

Maintaining constant glycemia and insulinemia

Increased fat consumption for energy purposes

Increase of the global caloric expenditure by increasing the specific dynamic action and the "metabolic work".

Has an anorectic effect

May be useful in counteracting symptoms of epilepsy that does not respond to medication, especially in children.

Disadvantages

Disadvantages of ketogenic diet

The ketogenic diet can also show several disadvantages, most of which depend on the levels of ketone bodies present in the blood:

Increased renal filtration and diuresis (excretion of ketone bodies and nitrogenous waste)

Tendency to dehydration

Increased workload of the kidneys

Possible toxic effect on kidneys by ketone bodies

Possible hypoglycemia

Possible hypotension

Keto-influenza or "keto-flu" in English; is a syndrome related to the body's poor adaptation after 2-3 days of starting the ketogenic diet. Includes:
Headaches
Fatigue
Dizziness
Mild nausea
Irritability.
In more sensitive individuals, increased chance of fainting (due to the previous two)
Increased tendency to:
Muscle cramps
Constipation
Sensation of heart palpitations
Increased workload of the liver, due to increased neoglucogenesis, processes of transamination and deamination
In the presence of intense and/or prolonged motor activity, muscle catabolism
It is unbalanced and tends to limit the intake of some nutrients, even very important ones
It can be particularly harmful for
Malnourished subjects such as, for example, subjects affected by eating disorders (DCA)
Type I diabetics
Pregnant and nursing mothers
Those already suffering from liver and/or kidney disease.
Scientific Updates
Carbohydrates: do they compromise health and promote mortality?

By carefully observing and comparing the list of advantages with the list of disadvantages, it seems that the ketogenic diet is not a real "godsend". In fact, it is a method that is contraindicated in several situations; it also requires a certain "individual sensitivity", or the use of analytical tools that ensure that it falls perfectly within the "ideal ketosis". It is undoubtedly a rather cumbersome and unspontaneous strategy. However, it is still widely used today in the context of weight loss and food therapy against chronic hyperglycemia. Scientific research suggests that, if used correctly, the ketogenic diet can not only be useful, but also remedy some of the damage caused by diets rich in carbohydrates (obesity, diabetes mellitus type 2, hypertriglyceridemia, etc).

PURE study by Dehghan et al., 2017

The PURE (Dehghan et al., 2017) is a prospective (or cohort) study that observed over 135,000 participants from 18 countries for many years. Excluding subjects with preexisting cardiovascular disease (except for diabetes), after a follow-up of 7.4 years from the beginning of observation, more than 10,000 deaths or cardiovascular events (such as heart attack and stroke) correlated with the parameters of the start of the study (socioeconomic factors, questionnaires on diet and motor activity); it was found that carbohydrate intake increased total mortality while lipids (indiscriminately saturated and unsaturated) decreased it. No link was noted between fat consumption and cardiovascular or other related mortality events, with the exception of saturated fat, which unexpectedly was associated with a lower risk of stroke.

The release of insulin caused by glucose intake and the activation of the corresponding signaling cascade may be considered the main reason that increasing carbohydrate intake promotes mortality. As shown by the high incidence of cancer in diabetics, hyperinsulinemia is a very important malignant growth factor.

Reduction of glucose absorption

From a therapeutic perspective, if carbohydrates are relevant factors in promoting mortality, not only reducing total intake but also inhibiting carbohydrate absorption and metabolism should prolong lifespan.

# Ketogenic Diet

# Acarbose

is an inhibitor of alpha-glucosidase, an intestinal enzyme that releases D-glucose from complex carbohydrates (especially starch). It has been used in the treatment of diabetics to limit the absorption of carbohydrates in the intestine since the 1980s. Consistent with the role of carbohydrates in compromising health, acarbose has been shown to extend lifespan in mice (Harrison et al., 2014)

Renal sodium-glucose co-transporter 2 (SGLT-2) inhibitors promote the removal of D-glucose from the blood through the urine. These newly developed inhibitors are used to treat diabetics. Potential effects on lifespan in organisms or humans have not yet been published but seem warranted.

The antidiabetic metformin, currently being investigated for lifespan extension (TAME study), reduces glucose production (gluconeogenesis) from the liver and causes a reduction in blood glucose.

Combination of nutrients

In mice, almost complete removal of carbohydrates (< 1%) to achieve a ketogenic diet improved life expectancy compared with a high-carbohydrate diet. On the other hand, Roberts et al., 2017 observed that replenishing even 10% of energy in simple sugars this positive effect vanishes. Replacing sugars with complex carbohydrates significantly improves the parameters; thus, it is the sugars that exert the worst effect. It has been shown that associating a diet high in fats with medium percentages of simple sugars gives negative results; however, the worst results were obtained by combining very high amounts of fats and sugars. In addition, extended lifespan of mice was noted by replacing nutritional protein with carbohydrates, independent of total calories (Solon-Biet et al., 2014). Taken together, these studies suggest that dietary sugar may be a very important, but not unique, limiting factor on rodent health.

# Ketogenic diet: is it worth it?

The PURE study has been criticized for manipulating the statistical effect of its findings. Specifically, the income- and geography-dependent nutritional habits of specific subgroups would not be applicable to Western high-income societies (which were nevertheless included in PURE). Indeed, Dehghan et al. (2017) did not analyze which specific source of carbohydrates (refined sugar/carbohydrates or whole grains) might contribute to the harmful effects of carbohydrates, and how income might influence the quality of dietary choices. However, additional elaboration on household income and wealth, as well as socioeconomic status in the respective country, was subsequently proposed, showing that these variables did not affect the main observations of the study in any way (Appendix, p. 34 of Dehghan et al., 2017).

Study Conclusion.

The research team of the PURE study believes that current nutritional recommendations, especially regarding refined carbohydrates and sugar, should be radically reconsidered. In addition, pharmacological options to simulate low-carbohydrate nutrition (i.e., without the need for actual reduction in carbohydrate intake) should be considered a useful and practical approach with respect to changes in nutritional habits for the general population.

Avoiding glucose intake through the diet and forcing the body to use the less convenient amino acids is a rather "questionable" strategy, because it intoxicates the whole organism, tends to fatigue liver and kidneys unnecessarily, makes the nervous system and muscles less efficient.

On the other hand, the potential serious negative effects of ketogenic diets are more limited than many believe; or rather, the ketogenic diet alone, in the short term, does not cause kidney failure, liver failure, reduction of basal metabolism and thyroid impairment, bone demineralization, etc.. What could happen in the long term is still the subject of studies; certainly, the ketogenic diet should not be understood as a definitive dietary strategy, especially given the contraindications it may have in certain situations.

However, there is no doubt that all this work, besides keeping glycemic-insulin levels low (responsible, together with caloric excess, for the deposit of fat), increases the amount of calories burned, stimulates the secretion of hormones and the production of metabolites that favor the disposal of fat and suppress appetite. For all these reasons, the "slimming" effectiveness of the ketogenic diet is all in all high.

The ketogenic diet works immediately but subjects the organism to a continuous and unhealthy stress. If badly designed, in particular when badly divided or excessively restrictive, the ketogenic diet must be abandoned and replaced with other less dangerous and equally effective dietary strategies.

Although it is also used in the treatment of epilepsy that does not respond adequately to drugs, in other contexts the ketogenic diet can be particularly harmful. In fact, it is one of the most popular "extreme" eating strategies in certain eating disorders (DCA). If performed by a subject affected by diabetes mellitus type 1 (even if actually there would be no reason for it), it requires a lot of attention and medical support, because it could have very serious consequences for health. Moreover, being strongly unbalanced, it can compromise the nutritional demand of the pregnant woman or the nurse.

The ketogenic diet is a dietary regimen that drastically reduces carbohydrates, while increasing proteins and especially fats. The purpose

main purpose of this imbalance in the proportions of macronutrients in the diet is to force the body to use fats as an energy source.

is to force the body to use fats as a source of energy. In the presence of carbohydrates, in fact, all the cells use their energy to

carry out their activities. But if these are reduced to a sufficiently low level they begin to use fats, all except the cells

nerve cells that do not have the ability to do so. A process called ketosis is then initiated, because it leads to the formation of molecules called ketone bodies, this time usable by the brain. Typically ketosis is reached after a couple of days with a daily amount of carbohydrates of about 20-50 grams, but these amounts can vary on an individual basis.

Ketosis is a toxic condition for the body, which provides for the disposal of ketone bodies through the renal pathway. Different is the pathological condition of metabolic acidosis, for example in the case of a complication of type 1 diabetes in which it comes to the accumulation of ketone bodies that give to the breath the characteristic odor of acetone. In children, ketosis can occur in the presence of high fever or strong emotional stress. This type of diet has a great impact on the organism, so much so that it was originally created as a diet recommended to reduce epileptic seizures in patients who did not respond to medication, especially in children.

Today the success of the ketogenic diet is mainly linked to its effectiveness in reducing weight, but it is important to emphasize that it is not an easy regime to follow. In fact, it is enough to "deviate" even a little in terms of carbohydrates to induce the body to block ketosis and to use again its preferred energy source: sugars. Those who have followed this diet - which is usually proposed for short periods of a few weeks - claim to have great energy once they reach the state of ketosis. But the days preceding this event are sometimes characterized by nausea, constipation, fatigue and breathing difficulties. Also
.there is no evidence that, in the long run, the results obtained are better and longer lasting than those achieved with a balanced diet.

The ketogenic diet is a dietary regimen that drastically reduces carbohydrates, while increasing proteins and especially fats. The purpose

main purpose of this imbalance of the proportions of macronutrients in the diet
is to force the body to use fats as a source of energy. In the presence of carbohydrates, in fact, all the cells use their energy to
carry out their activities. But if these are reduced to a sufficiently low level they begin to use fats, all except the cells

nerve cells that do not have the ability to do so. A process called ketosis is then initiated, because it leads to the formation of molecules called ketone bodies, this time usable by the brain. Typically ketosis is reached after a couple of days with a daily amount of carbohydrates of about 20-50 grams, but these amounts can vary on an individual basis.

Ketosis is a toxic condition for the body, which provides for the disposal of ketone bodies through the renal pathway. Different is the pathological condition of metabolic acidosis, for example in the case of a complication of type 1 diabetes in which it comes to the accumulation of ketone bodies that give to the breath the characteristic odor of acetone. In children, ketosis can occur in the presence of high fever or strong emotional stress. This type of diet has a great impact on the organism, so much so that it was originally created as a diet recommended to reduce epileptic seizures in patients who did not respond to medication, especially in children.

Today the success of the ketogenic diet is mainly linked to its effectiveness in reducing weight, but it is important to emphasize that it is not an easy regime to follow. In fact, it is enough to "deviate" even a little in terms of carbohydrates to induce the body to block ketosis and to use again its preferred energy source: sugars. Those who have followed this diet - which is usually proposed for short periods of a few weeks - claim to have great energy once they reach the state of ketosis. But the days preceding this event are sometimes characterized by nausea, constipation, fatigue and breathing difficulties. Also

.there is no evidence that, in the long run, the results obtained are better and more lasting than those achieved with a balanced diet.

The following indications have an EXCLUSIVE informative purpose and are not intended to replace the opinion of professional figures such as doctors, nutritionists or dieticians, whose intervention is necessary for the prescription and composition of PERSONALIZED food therapies.

Ketogenic Diet

# The Vandals Of The Ketogenic Diet

ATTENTION! With this article we will try to give an example of a diet based on the discharge of dietary carbohydrates and the parallel increase of ketone bodies in the blood. It is important to remember that we are referring exclusively to ONE ketogenic diet (in the generic sense) and not TO the ketogenic diet (a more or less specific method claimed by some professionals); this small clarification has the purpose of safeguarding the author of the article and my-personaltrainer.it from any claim on the intellectual property of the ketogenic diet or from any dispute of a conceptual-methodological nature.

The ketogenic diet is an unbalanced diet THAT NEEDS CONSTANT MONITORING BY THE MEDICAL SPECIALIST (through the analysis of ketone bodies, for example by testing the urinary pH). The ketogenic diet can be useful in the treatment of two totally different clinical conditions:

Overweight and metabolic disorders WITHOUT complications (kidneys and liver must be perfectly healthy)

Drug-resistant epilepsy, especially in children (see the article: Diet for epilepsy)

Below we will present an example of a slimming ketogenic diet and not a ketogenic diet to reduce the symptoms of epilepsy.

Reduction of simple and complex carbohydrates: foods containing carbohydrates must be totally eliminated (even if this is practically impossible). The portions of vegetables, which contain fructose, are maintained, thus determining the collapse of the percentage of complex carbohydrates in favor of simple ones (which however we remember are quantitatively very low). These nutrients represent the primary fuel of the body and reducing them "to a minimum" forces the body to dispose of excess fat reserves; in addition, carbohydrates are nutrients that significantly stimulate insulin (anabolic and fattening hormone), which is why their moderation should also assume an important metabolic significance.

Quantitative and percentage increase (therefore absolute) of fats, and only percentage of proteins, while maintaining a constant caloric intake: after eliminating carbohydrates, you should keep constant the portions of protein foods, increasing at the same time only the amount of foods high in fat (oils, oily seeds, fleshy oily fruits etc.). In theory, doing so compensates for the reduction

In theory, this compensates for the reduction in calories from the glucidic deficit thanks to the greater quantity of lipids. In practice, for obvious reasons of appetite (indeed, hunger!), it is necessary to

increase the portions and frequency of consumption of protein foods. Some people justify this "correction" by stating that more protein is useful to preserve lean mass. However, it should be noted that

many amino acids are glucogenic (they are converted into glucose by neoglucogenesis) and

have a metabolic action similar to dietary carbohydrates, partially negating the effect on lipolytic enzymes and ketone body production (see below). Moreover, in clinical practice, with the "calculator in hand", the menu of the ketogenic diet is NEVER normocaloric and always provides less energy than necessary. It would be better to try a well structured low-calorie balanced diet before trying such a mess.

Production of ketone bodies: the hepatic neoglucogenesis necessary to synthesize glucose (from certain amino acids and glycerol) is not fast enough to cover the daily glucose needs. In parallel, the oxidation of fats (closely related to and

dependent on glycolysis) "jams" and causes the accumulation of intermediate molecules (in my opinion, waste) called ketone bodies. These ketones, which at physiological concentrations are easily disposed of, in the ketogenic diet reach levels that are toxic to tissues.

Toxic does not necessarily mean poisonous, but rather "causing intoxication". This effect is clearly distinguishable by

reduction of appetite, i.e. the anorectic effect on the brain, although, like the heart, nervous tissue is also partially

capable of using ketone bodies for energy purposes.

The healthy organism is able to function even

with high blood quantities of ketone bodies, whose excess is eliminated (we do not know with how hard) by renal filtration. Obviously, people affected by certain diseases (defect of insulin secretion - typical of diabetes mellitus type 1 - renal failure - also triggered by advanced diabetes mellitus type 2 - liver failure etc.) have a very high risk to evolve in metabolic ketoacidosis risking coma or even death.

Perplexities about ketogenic diet

Personally, I consider the ketogenic diet a rather extreme method and I do not believe that its application can be defined DEONTHOLOGICALLY correct; however, as many clinicians demonstrate, sometimes it is necessary to act quickly on obesity to safeguard the health of the critical patient. For my part, I leave it to clinicians to evaluate and apply such a dietary regimen.

The PROTRACTED and DISCOMPENSED ketogenic diet (as we said above, in case of pre-existing disease) can promote the manifestation of:

Syndrome called "keto flu", that is a condition of generalized discomfort caused by the metabolic imbalance still not fully compensated by the body

Mood alterations and asthenia from physical activity

Acidosis or otherwise lowering of blood pH

Liver fatigue (even if not always measurable in the healthy subject)

Kidney fatigue (although not always measurable in healthy subjects)

Tendency to systemic dehydration

Illnesses of various kinds, such as hypoglycemia and low blood pressure that may begin with a blackout

Hypovitaminosis, salt and dietary fiber deficiency

Depletion of muscle tissue, especially in case of motor activity.

Note: It is curious to see how many of the above symptoms and clinical signs are common to marasmus (generalized malnutrition).

The ketogenic diet can not and should not be practiced for long and, if you decide to undertake it, it would be appropriate to remember that it is necessary to alternate periods of ketogenesis to days of restoration of glycogen stores. The body, especially the nervous tissue, needs about 180g/day of carbohydrates to function effectively and efficiently (although 50-100 grams should prevent ketoacidosis - Calloeay 1971), but this also means that following the ketogenic diet you will NEVER enjoy an OPTIMAL psycho-physical shape. On the other hand, many professionals who

advise to undertake the ketogenic diet suggest NOT to interrupt it because ketosis itself (which arises after a few days from the beginning) is fundamental to the good functioning of the system.

The ketogenic diet is not concerned with the ratio between complex carbohydrates and simple sugars, since carbohydrates are so scarce that their metabolic impact is almost marginal.

The ketogenic diet is NOT applicable to sportsmen and endurance athletes.

Useful supplements

The useful supplements in case of ketogenic diet are those that ensure the coverage of hydrosaline and vitamin needs. Many readers will think that in order to reach certain vitamin and salt quotas in ketogenic diet it is sufficient to increase the intake of vegetables, but unfortunately it is not so simple. Vegetables are rich in mineral salts and vitamins, as well as in fiber and anti-nutritional chelating molecules; therefore, by excessively increasing the intake of vegetables, the risk of malabsorption or partial absorption of nutrients (iron, calcium, vitamins, etc.) increases. Moreover, according to the principle of ketogenic diet, it is essential to reduce to the minimum the contribution of carbohydrates, however well present (even though in variable measure) in all vegetables.

The dosage of hydrosaline and vitamin supplements cannot be illustrated or suggested with precision because, given the heterogeneity of the products on the market, it would be an approximate and misleading indication to say the least. I suggest therefore to consult the label and to bring a MAXIMUM daily quantity of mineral salts and/or vitamins supplements equal to 50-80% of the total needs (personal opinion). It is also advisable to consult your doctor or pharmacist. It is also advisable to give preference to supplements containing minerals with alkalizing action, such as citrates (potassium citrate, magnesium citrate, sodium citrate) or bicarbonates (sodium bicarbonate, potassium bicarbonate, etc.).

Note: the ketogenic diet does not respect the principles of nutritional balance of the classical method and, by definition, is a NON-EQUILIBRATED dietary style since it is hypoglucidic, hyperlipidic and tends to be hyperproteic (in the context of the Mediterranean diet). It requires to disregard the calculation of needs, maintaining an intake of carbohydrates TOT not exceeding 50-100g/day even if, according to what some experts write, the lower the intake of carbohydrates, the greater the ketosis and the effectiveness of the system.

Ketogenic diet also suggests to provide a higher portion of unsaturated lipids than saturated ones. Protein intake can reach values decidedly out of the ordinary (up to and over 3g/kg of physiological weight), sometimes even reducing the amount of the "precious" total lipids.

The following indications are for information purposes ONLY and are not intended to replace the opinion of professional figures such as doctors, nutritionists or dieticians, whose intervention is necessary for the prescription and composition of PERSONALIZED food therapies.

ATTENTION! This article will try to give an example of diet based on the discharge of dietary carbohydrates and the parallel increase of ketone bodies in the blood. It's important to remember that we are referring exclusively to ONE ketogenic diet (in the generic sense) and not TO the ketogenic diet (a more or less specific method claimed by some professionals); this small clarification has the purpose of safeguarding the author of the article and my-personaltrainer.it from any claim on the intellectual property of the ketogenic diet or, why not, even from any disputes of a conceptual-methodological nature.

The ketogenic diet for muscle definition

The ketogenic diet for muscle definition in bodybuilding is an unbalanced diet that requires constant monitoring by the doctor.

CONSTANT MONITORING BY THE MEDICAL SPECIALIST; the ketogenic diet in body building is useful for weight loss but above all for muscle definition or CUTTING.

The ketogenic diet for muscle definition is essentially based on 3 concepts:

Carbohydrate reduction: contrary to a ketogenic diet for weight loss (applicable in case of overweight or obesity) or one for epilepsy (useful in case of drug resistance), the ketogenic diet for muscle definition must take into account the high intensity physical training of the body-builder. Without going into the details of training or energy physiology, in order to effectively stimulate strength and muscle hypertrophy it is ALWAYS necessary to maintain a dietary quota of sugars more significant than the diet for weight loss of a sedentary person; this means that: the portion of dietary carbohydrates in the ketogenic diet for muscle definition should be at the upper limits of the ketogenic diet for muscle definition.

This means that: the portion of dietary carbohydrates in the ketogenic diet for muscle definition should be at the upper limits of the range allowed for the application of this strategy. Excessively reducing carbohydrates in the ketogenic

excessive reduction of carbohydrates in the ketogenic diet for muscle definition would not be correct, since it would increase the risk of compromising physical efficiency during training and would promote the excessive catabolism of muscle proteins.

Parallel increase of proteins and fats in the diet: by reducing carbohydrates in the diet, in order not to excessively lower the total energy quota, it is essential to drastically increase the percentage and quantity of lipids and proteins (at least 3g/kg). Some claim that the ketogenic diet, especially when applied to bodybuilding, has a "metabolic-catabolic" effect which facilitates the depletion of adipose tissue even without reducing total energy, by simply replacing carbohydrates with fats and proteins. Personally, I think this is questionable to say the least.

Consequent production of ketone bodies and nitrogen groups: the ketogenic diet for muscle definition, like all ketogenic diets, induces the accumulation of ketone bodies and nitrogen groups. I

ketone bodies, intermediate between the anaerobic glycolysis and the Krebs cycle, are toxic to tissues and, while taking advantage of the

the reduction of the sense of appetite, especially in association with nitrogenous groups, have a negative impact on liver and kidney function. All these molecules facilitate body dehydration as they are strongly osmotic and responsible for the increased renal excretion of water and minerals (including calcium).

Negative aspects of the ketogenic diet

The ketogenic diet for muscle definition, especially if not properly monitored, can promote the appearance of:

Acidosis (very serious) or otherwise lowering of blood pH

Hepatic fatigue

Renal fatigue

Systemic dehydration

Various types of sickness, such as hypoglycemia and low blood pressure that can start with a black-out

Hypovitaminosis, salt and dietary fiber deficiency

Mood alterations and asthenia from physical activity

Depletion of muscle tissue

Increased renal excretion of calcium

Cholesterol intake up to 100% more than normal and saturated fat intake > 10% of total kcal or > 1/3 of total lipids.

Because of its toxicity and its marked catabolic effect, the ketogenic diet for definition should not be undertaken for long periods of time; moreover, if a bodybuilder decides to undertake it, he/she should find the right compromise between caloricity-diet breakdown and training. There are therefore multiple theories of application:

Placement of workouts ONLY on glucose recharge days (spaced by about 2 days of unloading)

If the training program is very demanding, it would be more appropriate to maintain a carbohydrate quota closer to the upper limit of the allowed range.

How many carbohydrates should you take?

THE HUMAN BODY REQUIRES ABOUT 180G/DAY OF CARBOHYDRATES TO ENSURE EFFICIENT BRAIN FUNCTION EVEN IN THE LONG TERM

(FAO, 1980), ALTHOUGH IT HAS ALREADY BEEN DEMONSTRATED THAT ONLY 50-100G/DIE OF CARBOHYDRATES SHOULD BE SUFFICIENT TO PREVENT KETOSIS (CALLOEAY 1971).

Assuming that 180g/day represents a suitable preventive quota in a diet of 1800kcal (CHO at 37.5%, against 55-65% of a balanced diet), and taking the maximum value of the safety range proposed above (100g/day - CHO at 20.8%) it is possible to define that:under conditions

of sedentariness, a subject who assumes 1800kcal could MAINTAIN nervous function by reducing carbohydrates up to 37.5%, and further lower them up to 20.8% WITHOUT INCREASING THE RISK OF CHETOACIDOSIS.

... AND IN THE BODY-BUILDER WHO ALSO PRACTICES INTENSE WORKOUTS?

Hard to say, although we could hypothesize a specific method; so:

Estimate the ketogenic of the sedentary on the maximum values of the range (100g CHO, or 20.8%kcal TOT)

Sum of energy expenditure of each workout, e.g. 300kcal, covered by mixed maltodextrin and branched-chain amino acid supplements.

NB. The ketogenic diet is not concerned with the ratio of complex sugars to simple sugars, since carbohydrates are so scarce that their metabolic impact assumes an absolutely marginal value.

The methods for the preparation of a ketogenic diet are many, as many as the variables to be taken into account in each individual outpatient case; below will be

an example of a ketogenic diet for muscle definition will be proposed below, with the objective of maintaining a stable food COMPENSATION of the glucidic portion (at least 100g of CHO/day + maltodextrin supplements in training), making it necessary to have only one
only one day of weekly recharge.
NB.The ketogenic diet is NOT applicable, as counterproductive and dangerous, to sportsmen or endurance/resistance athletes.
Useful supplements
The supplements useful in case of ketogenic diet are those that ensure the coverage of hydrosaline and vitamin needs; in the event that it is necessary to meet a higher energy expenditure than normal, it may be good practice to consume a supplement based on maltodextrin and branched chain amino acids. Some consider it essential to associate to the ketogenic cycles a phase of dietary supplementation of creatine (if constant, about 3g / day), in order to promote the accumulation in the muscles and accentuate the anaerobic metabolism LACTIC sparing tissue glycogen.
NB. If the subject presents a significant increase in blood cholesterol, it is possible to replace part of the animal foods with supplements based on protein powder (possibly soy), in order to contain the exogenous intake of this lipid.

The term diabetic ketoacidosis refers to a dreaded acute complication of type 1 diabetes mellitus, although more rarely it can also affect patients with type 2 diabetes.

The condition develops when the body is no longer able to produce sufficient insulin, a molecule that plays a key role in allowing sugar to pass from the blood to muscles and other tissues; without the ability to use sugar as fuel, cells begin to rely on fat to survive, but this metabolic change results in the production and accumulation of ketones in the blood.

Ketoacidosis presents itself with the appearance of

hyperglycemia

increased circulating ketones,

which in turn are responsible for characteristic symptoms such as:

increased thirst and frequency of urination,

malaise,

fruity breath,

increased frequency of breathing

fatigue,

confusion,

fainting.

Diagnosis is often based on blood tests, while treatment involves rehydrating the patient and administering insulin.

## Causes

Type 1 diabetes is based on the (total or partial) deficiency of insulin, a hormone whose main task is to allow glucose, which travels freely in the bloodstream, to be stored within all the cells of our body to be then used in a more or less immediate way.

When insulin is lacking, a state of chronic hyperglycemia ensues: glucose, which can no longer be transferred within the cells, persists in the peripheral blood and its levels in the blood (glycemia) rise dangerously.

In order to avoid this situation, the diabetic patient is instructed by the diabetologist to perform regular insulin administrations, so as to allow the correct sugar metabolism to take place.

In the absence of sugar, some cells have the urgent need to find an alternative energy source and this is particularly true for the cells of the nervous system.

true for the cells of the central nervous system: the source that these cells tend to use is represented by fatty acids. However, the use of fats has as a consequence the production and above all

the accumulation of characteristic waste products, called "ketone bodies".

The ketone bodies are released into the blood, with the consequence of lowering the pH (acidification of the blood).

At the same time, blood glucose levels are kept high, but the inability of the cell to take it from the blood activates hyperglycemic mechanisms aimed at releasing glucose from the body's reserves, a process that leads to a further rise in blood glucose levels, thus triggering and feeding a dangerous vicious circle.

Risk Factors

Every type 1 diabetic patient is exposed to the risk of developing diabetic ketoacidosis and, although it is not always possible to trace the cause, among the factors capable of triggering the process we can recall

presence of infection, such as flu or a urinary tract infection (cystitis, for example)
forgetfulness and errors in the administration of insulin,
injury or surgery,
certain medications (such as cortisone),
excess alcohol,
consumption of substances of abuse,
pregnancy,

menstrual flow.

Symptoms
At the clinical level, the characteristic sign of the patient suffering from ketoacidosis is represented by the acetonic or fruity breath, due to the elimination of acetone produced by the catabolism of ketone bodies (in a similar way, but with different order of magnitude, of what happens in the ketosis of children).
Clinical symptoms are represented by:
Polyuria, which is an increase in 24-hour urine elimination above 2 liters per day. It is a typical condition in fact of type 1 diabetes, independently from ketoacidosis, but in this condition tends to become more pronounced.
Polydipsia, or increased sense of thirst. It is obviously a direct consequence of polyuria.
Hypotension (lowering of blood pressure), may occur in response to excessive fluid loss if this is not adequately compensated.
Nausea and vomiting.
Loss of appetite.
Generalized agitation.

Tachypnea (increased rate of breathing).

Loss of attention or simply drowsiness, which can therefore often go unnoticed, especially if we talk about ketoacidosis in a child.

Fever may also sometimes appear, which in some cases may be due to a real underlying infection that may be the trigger of the condition.

We must remember that type 1 diabetes often arises at a young age, a characteristic that differentiates it from type 2 diabetes, typical of more advanced ages.

Diabetic ketoacidosis can sometimes be the first form of acute manifestation of a type 1 diabetes still undiagnosed especially in children, where often these symptoms can be confused or even underestimated.

Diagnosis

The diagnosis is usually based on the earliest identification of the characteristic symptoms, so as to be able to stop the imbalance in time and avoid more serious sequelae.

From the laboratory point of view the diagnosis is based on the finding of:

hyperglycemia, which tends to rise further and further in view of the activation of hyperglycemic mechanisms that cells activate in glucose deficiency within them;

ketone bodies, as well as a lowering of the pH related to the presence of the latter; the pH is monitored in the hospital through a particular invasive test called arterial blood gas analysis (or EGA).

Care

Since the first risk for the patient with ketoacidosis is represented by dehydration and subsequent hypotension, the initial therapy must be based on adequate rehydration of the patient, a process during which it is important to control the electrolyte balance, in order to avoid sudden changes in concentration (especially of sodium and potassium).

The basic therapy is therefore aimed at an adequate metabolic compensation of glucose; this condition, in a patient suffering from type 1 diabetes mellitus and therefore condemned for life to produce a lower than normal amount of insulin, is obviously linked to the administration of exogenous insulin.

Administering insulin from outside allows glucose to enter the cell, which is able to use it as a primary energy source avoiding the need to resort to alternative energy substrates and their harmful waste products; this is especially true for brain cells.

The entry of sugars inside the cells allows at the same time to lower the state of chronic hyperglycemia.

In the patient with already diagnosed diabetes, especially if he/she is a child, the prevention of a risky condition such as diabetic ketoacidosis can be performed only through a careful control of glycemic values and of the doses of insulin necessary to maintain the correct balance. Even in case of fasting it is still essential to maintain the insulin compensation, since fasting facilitates the onset of a ketogenic mechanism (going to use always and in any case the alternative reserves based on fatty acids).

If obviously the patient, child or not, does not know he has diabetes, being able to prevent ketoacidosis is more complex, because often ketoacidosis can be the first form of manifestation. However, it is of fundamental importance to always monitor signs and symptoms of alarm such as
drowsiness
acetonic breath
alterations of breathing
or heart rate.

We talk about it more and more often online: the ketogenic diet is praised by many, criticized by others, but what are really its benefits and contraindications? When can it be useful and which foods can be consumed?

The ketogenic diet seems to be the latest trend in terms of wellness and weight loss, but, as with any type of diet, it is always good to fully understand how it works, its impact on the body and how to integrate it into your lifestyle, preferably with the support of a nutrition specialist.

In a nutshell, what is the ketogenic diet? It is a different balance of the so-called MACROS, the macronutrients we consume daily: by drastically decreasing the intake of carbohydrates, considered the "gasoline" of the body, and moderately increasing the consumption of proteins and especially fats, the body is forced to work differently, burning lipids instead of sugar. To speak simply of a LOW-CARB approach, therefore, is a bit reductive.

This process is called ketosis and, as you can easily imagine, if properly managed, it can lead to a considerable loss of weight and fat mass.

We want to give you some indication of the mechanisms behind ketosis, the foods allowed and those to be eliminated according to this food plan and the potential pros and cons of adopting it.

The process of ketosis, how it works and when it is useful

Making some historical notes of medical literature, we talk about ketogenic diet at a medical level in relation to particular pathologies: some decades ago correlations were discovered between this diet and the control of pathologies such as epilepsy in childhood.

Another clinical condition which has been cured, in the course of time, through the induction of dietary ketosis is diabetes, as the diabetic patient is already struggling with a difficult management of sugars. Tests have even been done on patients affected by mental disorders, or by serious degenerative conditions such as Parkinson's and Alzheimer's, which in many cases would have benefited from a ketogenic food plan.

It is always good to make a clear distinction between a physiological ketosis, voluntarily induced in a healthy person followed by a nutritionist for weight loss or therapeutic purposes, and the DIABETIC KETOACIDOSIS, which is instead a serious disease that affects precisely people with diabetes, or even the ketosis developed by people suffering from eating disorders as a reaction to too restrictive regimens.

Scientifically speaking, this process occurs when the body does not have enough carbohydrates to use as fuel and, therefore, begins to draw energy from fat. Nerve cells, however, do not have this capacity: that's why ketosis is triggered, that is the formation of KETONIC BODIES, particular molecules that can be used also by nerve cells in the brain.

## The three phases of the keto diet

Typically, we talk about a 3-phase approach:
in the first phase, of "activation", which lasts about 48-72 hours, the reduction of carbohydrates causes the subject to enter ketosis;
the second phase, of "attack", which in order to have slimming effects should last a minimum of 14 days, is that linked to the consumption of fat mass, because the body, deprived of its natural fuel, i.e. sugar, begins to attack the lipid reserves;
the third phase is the one defined "mitigated", that is a slow transition to a more traditional and balanced eating style, but always with a careful eye on glycemic indexes and not to exceed with carbohydrates, for an effective maintenance.
Keto diet, foods: what to eat?
But what can we put on the table if we are trying the keto diet? As mentioned above, very few carbohydrates with a low glycemic index, moderate amounts of protein and a substantial dose of fats, the good ones of course.

You will be amazed at how many hidden sugars there are even in the most unthinkable foods and often associated with other macronutrients. One example? Legumes, traditionally considered a great source of vegetable proteins, are also rich in carbohydrates, that's why they should not be consumed often.

Among vegetables, no to potatoes and other tubers, no to fruits and vegetables with a few low-sugar exceptions, such as zucchini, broccoli, cucumbers, blueberries and raspberries.

For the protein component, yes to white meat, eggs, fish - better if caught and not farmed - Greek yogurt and natural skyr without added sugars, cheese, mushrooms and shellfish.

Among the best fats are avocado, coconut oil that you can find on our website, nuts and seeds, olive oil and clarified butter.

Not even the shadow of sweets or sweeteners, even honey is forbidden, at most natural stevia is allowed.

There are many recipes, by now, dedicated to those who are struggling with keto, some of them so tasty that they do not make you regret the traditional dishes, but it is certainly a great challenge to continue this dietary style for a long time without incurring in temptations and excesses. The brain, in fact, tends to want what it lacks, leading physiologically to crave sugar.

## The pros of the ketogenic diet

Among the pros recognized by most, even by some celebrities who have declared to have adopted this dietary scheme, there is the possibility to lose not only weight but also localized fat, burning accumulations and excesses.

Besides this factor - aesthetic for many but also of health for all those who suffer from pathologies related to overweight - there is also a chemical component. Ketosis, in fact, would favor the stabilization of the mood, no longer "influenced" by glycemic fluctuations. Those who manage to overcome the first phase, in fact, often claim to feel full of energy, motivated and cheerful.

The hormones that help stabilize mood also serve to promote an anorectic effect, that is a natural limitation of appetite, which obviously helps if the goal is weight loss.

The cons of the ketogenic diet

Among the major cons, the main one is almost a triviality: glucose is essential for the survival of any healthy organism. Cutting out carbohydrates completely for a long period of time, therefore, can bring serious consequences on a psycho-physical level.

The second cons is also a very strong consideration: ketosis is, in itself, a toxic consideration for the human body, an abnormality. The molecules called ketones, as waste, are eliminated through the kidneys and the liver, forced therefore to an onerous work of disposal.

It increases, for this reason, the risk of dehydration, as well as not meeting the needs in terms of micronutrients, in particular calcium and vitamins, and fiber.

These negative effects are enhanced by the fact that those who seek rapid weight loss through the ketogenic diet usually also combine it with sports activity. Exercise makes the body need glucose even more, thus exacerbating the mechanisms and criticalities we have described.

We suggest, therefore, as for any other decision concerning one's health, to always consult a professional before heavily modifying one's eating behavior, especially in the presence of particular conditions and previous pathologies.

# WHAT IS AN EXAMPLE OF KETOGENIC DIET AND WHEN TO FOLLOW IT

## WHAT IS IT AND HOW IS STRUCTURED AN EXAMPLE OF KETOGENIC DIET

We often hear about ketogenic diet simply as a high-protein diet, but actually the amount of nutrients in this type of diet are different from the high-protein diet.

In fact, a ketogenic diet involves the intake of carbohydrates in low quantities, proteins in normal quantities and a high amount of fats. In a high protein diet carbohydrates are even lower while proteins are much higher than the recommended daily quantity. Fats on the other hand are kept in the normal range.

So, if you wanted to follow an example of ketogenic diet what would be the basic mechanism that would make you lose weight? Let's see it together.

## HOW DO YOU LOSE WEIGHT ON THE KETOGENIC DIET?

This diet takes its name from the process of ketosis: our body when it doesn't have enough sugars to transform into energy begins to draw on fat reserves by transforming them into sugars. For this reason, carbohydrates must remain low, because by consuming more our body would not draw on body fat.

The signal that you have entered the ketosis phase is the weight loss, from that moment on it is therefore necessary to continue following the diet in order not to stop or slow down this process and therefore having to start all over again.

Here then is an example of ketogenic diet that will show you the foods allowed, for doses or other indications we always recommend you to consult a nutritionist.

## EXAMPLE OF KETOGENIC DIET: FOODS AND SCHEME TO FOLLOW

As for any other type of diet, also for ketogenic diet the foods and their doses should be customized according to the patient's state of health and tastes.

However here is a general list of foods which are allowed in ketogenic diet:

Carbohydrates: to be preferred are whole grains, which release sugars more slowly avoiding glycemic peaks and reducing the sense of hunger. Particularly recommended is oats.

Protein: all types of proteins are allowed, both animal and vegetable, including dairy products, to be consumed in smaller quantities than other sources of protein.

Fats: yes, but the good ones, therefore from dried fruit or extra virgin olive oil.

Vegetables: almost all are allowed and can be consumed both raw and cooked.

## WHAT IS THE ROLE OF HYDRATION?

During a ketogenic diet, the recommended number of liters of water is 2. However, in order to help the body to purify itself and to favor the activity of bowels, it is possible to take decoctions or natural herbal teas. Here are some advices:

Herbal teas: to be preferred are herbal teas made of chamomile, lemon balm and fennel which have a detoxifying power and help digestion. Examples are the herbal teas Erbo Ritual Detox and Relax herbal tea of the same line.

Decoctions: decoctions are concentrated vegetal extracts in liquid form which are then diluted with water. Precisely because of their high concentration they have a much higher draining power than herbal teas. You can also find them in the Tisanoreica kits together with meals and supplements that will help you in your diet.

that will help you in your ketogenic diet. Some examples are the Tisanoreica Intensive Kit or the Stabilization Kit from the same line. If, on the other hand, you are looking for products that will help you fight cellulite and take care of your body, you can try the Tisanoreica Body in Shape kit.

## TO WHOM IS A KETOGENIC DIET RECOMMENDED?

A ketogenic diet should be followed for a limited period of time and can be followed by all healthy adult individuals. In particular, this diet has shown particular benefits for:

People with type 2 diabetes

Treatment of obesity

People who suffer from migraine

People suffering from epilepsy

Individuals who suffer from metabolic syndrome

On the other hand, this diet cannot be followed by:

People who have kidney, liver and heart diseases

Pregnant women

People who suffer from type 1 diabetes

Young people who are still developing and growing

Contact us to have some more examples of ketogenic diets or to know all the products of the Tisanoreica line which can help you to do it.

# Ketogenic Diet

Ketogenic Diet

Lightning Source UK Ltd.
Milton Keynes UK
UKHW02063603O621
384863UK00011B/1292